# THIS JOURNAL BELONGS TO:

# CHILD'S GOALS

## SPEECH & COMMUNICATION GOALS

## SOCIAL SKILLS GOALS

## SENSORY GOALS

# ACTIVITY IDEAS

## FINE MOTOR ACTIVITIES

## VESTIBULAR/PROPRIOCEPTIVE

## TACTILE

## VISUAL

## AUDITORY

## ORAL

**NOTES:**

# MILESTONE TRACKER

| DATE: | |
|---|---|
| | |
| | |
| | |
| | |
| | |
| | |
| | |
| | |
| | |
| | |
| | |
| | |
| | |
| | |
| | |
| | |
| | |
| | |
| | |
| | |
| | |
| | |
| | |
| | |
| | |
| | |
| | |
| | |
| | |
| | |
| | |
| | |

# BOOKS TO READ TOGETHER

| BOOK TITLE | ✓ | BOOK TITLE | ✓ |
|---|---|---|---|
| | | | |
| | | | |
| | | | |
| | | | |
| | | | |
| | | | |
| | | | |
| | | | |
| | | | |
| | | | |
| | | | |
| | | | |
| | | | |
| | | | |
| | | | |
| | | | |
| | | | |
| | | | |
| | | | |
| | | | |
| | | | |
| | | | |

# WEEK 1 ACTIVITIES:

**MONDAY**

**TUESDAY**

**WEDNESDAY**

**THURSDAY**

**FRIDAY**

**SATURDAY**

**SUNDAY**

# WEEK 1:

**WEEK OF:** _____

### SPEECH & COMMUNICATION

### SENSORY & O.T.

### VESTIBULAR

### TACTILE

### ORAL MOTOR

| | |
|---|---|
| **MON** | |
| **TUE** | |
| **WED** | |
| **THUR** | |
| **FRI** | |
| **SAT** | |
| **SUN** | |

# WEEK 1:

## FINE MOTOR

## VISUAL

## AUDITORY

## THIS WEEK'S CHALLENGES

## SOCIAL SKILLS

## THIS WEEK'S HIGHLIGHTS

## OUR FAVORITE MOMENT

# WEEKLY APPOINTMENTS

**WEEK OF:** _____

| MON |
| --- |

_____
_____
_____
_____
_____

| TUE |
| --- |

_____
_____
_____
_____

| WED |
| --- |

_____
_____
_____
_____

| THU |
| --- |

_____
_____
_____
_____

# WEEKLY APPOINTMENTS

**WEEK OF:** _____

| FRI |
|-----|

| SAT |
|-----|

| SUN |
|-----|

# WEEKLY REFLECTION

## Weekly Challenges

## Weekly Accomplishments

## Favorite Moment of the Week

## NOTES

# WEEK 2 ACTIVITIES:

**MONDAY**

**TUESDAY**

**WEDNESDAY**

**THURSDAY**

**FRIDAY**

**SATURDAY**

**SUNDAY**

# WEEK 2:

**WEEK OF:** _____

## SPEECH & COMMUNICATION

## SENSORY & O.T.

## VESTIBULAR

## TACTILE

## ORAL MOTOR

| | |
|---|---|
| MON | |
| TUE | |
| WED | |
| THUR | |
| FRI | |
| SAT | |
| SUN | |

# WEEK 2:

## FINE MOTOR

## VISUAL

## AUDITORY

## THIS WEEK'S CHALLENGES

## SOCIAL SKILLS

## THIS WEEK'S HIGHLIGHTS

## OUR FAVORITE MOMENT

# WEEKLY APPOINTMENTS

**WEEK OF:** _____

| MON |
| --- |

_____
_____
_____
_____
_____

| TUE |
| --- |

_____
_____
_____
_____
_____

| WED |
| --- |

_____
_____
_____
_____

| THU |
| --- |

_____
_____
_____
_____

# WEEKLY APPOINTMENTS

**WEEK OF:** _____

FRI

SAT

SUN

# WEEKLY REFLECTION

## Weekly Challenges

## Weekly Accomplishments

## Favorite Moment of the Week

## NOTES

# WEEK 3 ACTIVITIES:

**MONDAY**

**TUESDAY**

**WEDNESDAY**

**THURSDAY**

**FRIDAY**

**SATURDAY**

**SUNDAY**

# WEEK 3:

**WEEK OF:** _____

## SPEECH & COMMUNICATION

## SENSORY & O.T.

## VESTIBULAR

## TACTILE

## ORAL MOTOR

| | MON |
|---|---|
| | TUE |
| | WED |
| | THUR |
| | FRI |
| | SAT |
| | SUN |

# WEEK 3:

## FINE MOTOR

## VISUAL

## AUDITORY

## THIS WEEK'S CHALLENGES

## THIS WEEK'S HIGHLIGHTS

## SOCIAL SKILLS

## OUR FAVORITE MOMENT

# WEEKLY APPOINTMENTS

**WEEK OF:** _____

MON

_____
_____
_____
_____
_____

TUE

_____
_____
_____
_____
_____

WED

_____
_____
_____
_____
_____

THU

_____
_____
_____
_____

# WEEKLY APPOINTMENTS

**WEEK OF:** _____

FRI

SAT

SUN

# WEEKLY REFLECTION

## Weekly Challenges

## Weekly Accomplishments

## Favorite Moment of the Week

## NOTES

# WEEK 4 ACTIVITIES:

**MONDAY**

**TUESDAY**

**WEDNESDAY**

**THURSDAY**

**FRIDAY**

**SATURDAY**

**SUNDAY**

# WEEK 4:

**WEEK OF:** _____

### SPEECH & COMMUNICATION

### SENSORY & O.T.

### VESTIBULAR

### TACTILE

### ORAL MOTOR

| | |
|---|---|
| **MON** | |
| **TUE** | |
| **WED** | |
| **THUR** | |
| **FRI** | |
| **SAT** | |
| **SUN** | |

# WEEK 4:

## FINE MOTOR

## VISUAL

## AUDITORY

## THIS WEEK'S CHALLENGES

## SOCIAL SKILLS

## THIS WEEK'S HIGHLIGHTS

## OUR FAVORITE MOMENT

# WEEKLY APPOINTMENTS

**WEEK OF:** _____

MON

TUE

WED

THU

# WEEKLY APPOINTMENTS

**WEEK OF:** _____

**FRI**

**SAT**

**SUN**

# WEEKLY REFLECTION

## Weekly Challenges

## Weekly Accomplishments

## Favorite Moment of the Week

## NOTES

# WEEK 5 ACTIVITIES:

**MONDAY**

**TUESDAY**

**WEDNESDAY**

**THURSDAY**

**FRIDAY**

**SATURDAY**

**SUNDAY**

# WEEK 5:

**WEEK OF:** _____

### SPEECH & COMMUNICATION

### SENSORY & O.T.

### VESTIBULAR

### TACTILE

### ORAL MOTOR

| | |
|---|---|
| **MON** | |
| **TUE** | |
| **WED** | |
| **THUR** | |
| **FRI** | |
| **SAT** | |
| **SUN** | |

# WEEK 5:

## FINE MOTOR

## VISUAL

## AUDITORY

## THIS WEEK'S CHALLENGES

## SOCIAL SKILLS

## THIS WEEK'S HIGHLIGHTS

## OUR FAVORITE MOMENT

# WEEKLY APPOINTMENTS

**WEEK OF:** _____

MON

TUE

WED

THU

# WEEKLY APPOINTMENTS

**WEEK OF:** _____

FRI

SAT

SUN

# WEEKLY REFLECTION

## Weekly Challenges

## Weekly Accomplishments

## Favorite Moment of the Week

## NOTES

# WEEK 6 ACTIVITIES:

**MONDAY**

**TUESDAY**

**WEDNESDAY**

**THURSDAY**

**FRIDAY**

**SATURDAY**

**SUNDAY**

# WEEK 6:

**WEEK OF:** _____

### SPEECH & COMMUNICATION

### SENSORY & O.T.

### VESTIBULAR

### TACTILE

### ORAL MOTOR

| | MON |
|---|---|
| | TUE |
| | WED |
| | THUR |
| | FRI |
| | SAT |
| | SUN |

# WEEK 6:

## FINE MOTOR

## VISUAL

## AUDITORY

## THIS WEEK'S CHALLENGES

## THIS WEEK'S HIGHLIGHTS

## SOCIAL SKILLS

## OUR FAVORITE MOMENT

# WEEKLY APPOINTMENTS

**WEEK OF:** _____

### MON

_____
_____
_____
_____
_____

### TUE

_____
_____
_____
_____

### WED

_____
_____
_____
_____

### THU

_____
_____
_____
_____

# WEEKLY APPOINTMENTS

**WEEK OF:** _____

| FRI |
|-----|

| SAT |
|-----|

| SUN |
|-----|

# WEEKLY REFLECTION

## Weekly Challenges

## Weekly Accomplishments

## Favorite Moment of the Week

## NOTES

# WEEK 7 ACTIVITIES:

MONDAY

TUESDAY

WEDNESDAY

THURSDAY

FRIDAY

SATURDAY

SUNDAY

# WEEK 7:

**WEEK OF:** _____

## SPEECH & COMMUNICATION

## SENSORY & O.T.

## VESTIBULAR

## TACTILE

## ORAL MOTOR

| MON | |
| --- | --- |
| TUE | |
| WED | |
| THUR | |
| FRI | |
| SAT | |
| SUN | |

# WEEK 7:

## FINE MOTOR

## VISUAL

## AUDITORY

## THIS WEEK'S CHALLENGES

## SOCIAL SKILLS

## THIS WEEK'S HIGHLIGHTS

## OUR FAVORITE MOMENT

# WEEKLY APPOINTMENTS

**WEEK OF:** _____

MON

_____
_____
_____
_____
_____

TUE

_____
_____
_____
_____
_____

WED

_____
_____
_____
_____
_____

THU

_____
_____
_____
_____
_____

# WEEKLY APPOINTMENTS

**WEEK OF:** _____

FRI

SAT

SUN

# WEEKLY REFLECTION

## Weekly Challenges

## Weekly Accomplishments

## Favorite Moment of the Week

## NOTES

# WEEK 8 ACTIVITIES:

**MONDAY**

**TUESDAY**

**WEDNESDAY**

**THURSDAY**

**FRIDAY**

**SATURDAY**

**SUNDAY**

# WEEK 8:

**WEEK OF:** _____

### SPEECH & COMMUNICATION

### SENSORY & O.T.

### VESTIBULAR

### TACTILE

### ORAL MOTOR

| | |
|---|---|
| **MON** | |
| **TUE** | |
| **WED** | |
| **THUR** | |
| **FRI** | |
| **SAT** | |
| **SUN** | |

# WEEK 8:

## FINE MOTOR

## VISUAL

## AUDITORY

## THIS WEEK'S CHALLENGES

## SOCIAL SKILLS

## THIS WEEK'S HIGHLIGHTS

## OUR FAVORITE MOMENT

# WEEKLY APPOINTMENTS

**WEEK OF:** _____

### MON

_____
_____
_____
_____
_____

### TUE

_____
_____
_____
_____
_____

### WED

_____
_____
_____
_____
_____

### THU

_____
_____
_____
_____
_____

# WEEKLY APPOINTMENTS

**WEEK OF:** _____

FRI

SAT

SUN

# WEEKLY REFLECTION

## Weekly Challenges

## Weekly Accomplishments

## Favorite Moment of the Week

## NOTES

# WEEK 9 ACTIVITIES:

**MONDAY**

**TUESDAY**

**WEDNESDAY**

**THURSDAY**

**FRIDAY**

**SATURDAY**

**SUNDAY**

# WEEK 9:

**WEEK OF:** _____

## SPEECH & COMMUNICATION

## SENSORY & O.T.

## VESTIBULAR

## TACTILE

## ORAL MOTOR

| MON | |
| --- | --- |
| TUE | |
| WED | |
| THUR | |
| FRI | |
| SAT | |
| SUN | |

# WEEK 9:

## FINE MOTOR

## VISUAL

## AUDITORY

## THIS WEEK'S CHALLENGES

## SOCIAL SKILLS

## THIS WEEK'S HIGHLIGHTS

## OUR FAVORITE MOMENT

# WEEKLY APPOINTMENTS

**WEEK OF:** _____

MON

TUE

WED

THU

# WEEKLY APPOINTMENTS

**WEEK OF:** _____

| FRI |
| --- |

| SAT |
| --- |

| SUN |
| --- |

# WEEKLY REFLECTION

Weekly Challenges

Weekly Accomplishments

Favorite Moment of the Week

## NOTES

# WEEK 10 ACTIVITIES:

**MONDAY**

**TUESDAY**

**WEDNESDAY**

**THURSDAY**

**FRIDAY**

**SATURDAY**

**SUNDAY**

# WEEK 10:

**WEEK OF:** _____

### SPEECH & COMMUNICATION

### SENSORY & O.T.

### VESTIBULAR

### TACTILE

### ORAL MOTOR

| MON | |
|-----|---|
| TUE | |
| WED | |
| THUR | |
| FRI | |
| SAT | |
| SUN | |

# WEEK 10:

## FINE MOTOR

## VISUAL

## AUDITORY

## THIS WEEK'S CHALLENGES

## THIS WEEK'S HIGHLIGHTS

## SOCIAL SKILLS

## OUR FAVORITE MOMENT

# WEEKLY APPOINTMENTS

**WEEK OF:** _____

| MON |
| --- |

_____
_____
_____
_____
_____

| TUE |
| --- |

_____
_____
_____
_____

| WED |
| --- |

_____
_____
_____
_____

| THU |
| --- |

_____
_____
_____
_____

# WEEKLY APPOINTMENTS

**WEEK OF:** _____

| FRI |
|-----|

| SAT |
|-----|

| SUN |
|-----|

# WEEKLY REFLECTION

## Weekly Challenges

## Weekly Accomplishments

## Favorite Moment of the Week

## NOTES

# WEEK 11 ACTIVITIES:

**MONDAY**

**TUESDAY**

**WEDNESDAY**

**THURSDAY**

**FRIDAY**

**SATURDAY**

**SUNDAY**

# WEEK 11:

**WEEK OF:** _____

### SPEECH & COMMUNICATION

### SENSORY & O.T.

### VESTIBULAR

### TACTILE

### ORAL MOTOR

MON

TUE

WED

THUR

FRI

SAT

SUN

# WEEK 11:

## FINE MOTOR

## VISUAL

## AUDITORY

## THIS WEEK'S CHALLENGES

## THIS WEEK'S HIGHLIGHTS

## SOCIAL SKILLS

## OUR FAVORITE MOMENT

# WEEKLY APPOINTMENTS

**WEEK OF:** _____

MON

TUE

WED

THU

# WEEKLY APPOINTMENTS

**WEEK OF:** _____

FRI

SAT

SUN

# WEEKLY REFLECTION

## Weekly Challenges

## Weekly Accomplishments

## Favorite Moment of the Week

## NOTES

# WEEK 12 ACTIVITIES:

**MONDAY**

**TUESDAY**

**WEDNESDAY**

**THURSDAY**

**FRIDAY**

**SATURDAY**

**SUNDAY**

# WEEK 12:

**WEEK OF:** _____

## SPEECH & COMMUNICATION

## SENSORY & O.T.

## VESTIBULAR

## TACTILE

## ORAL MOTOR

| MON | |
| --- | --- |
| TUE | |
| WED | |
| THUR | |
| FRI | |
| SAT | |
| SUN | |

# WEEK 12:

## FINE MOTOR

## VISUAL

## AUDITORY

## THIS WEEK'S CHALLENGES

## SOCIAL SKILLS

## THIS WEEK'S HIGHLIGHTS

## OUR FAVORITE MOMENT

# WEEKLY APPOINTMENTS

**WEEK OF:** _____

MON

TUE

WED

THU

# WEEKLY APPOINTMENTS

**WEEK OF:** _____

FRI

SAT

SUN

# WEEKLY REFLECTION

_____

_____

_____

_____

_____

_____

_____

_____

_____

_____

_____

_____

_____

_____

_____

_____

_____

_____

_____

_____

| Weekly Challenges |
| --- |
| |

| Weekly Accomplishments |
| --- |
| |

| Favorite Moment of the Week |
| --- |
| |

| **NOTES** |
| --- |
| |

# WEEK 13 ACTIVITIES:

**MONDAY**

**TUESDAY**

**WEDNESDAY**

**THURSDAY**

**FRIDAY**

**SATURDAY**

**SUNDAY**

# WEEK 13:

**WEEK OF:** _____

## SPEECH & COMMUNICATION

## SENSORY & O.T.

## VESTIBULAR

## TACTILE

## ORAL MOTOR

| | |
|---|---|
| MON | |
| TUE | |
| WED | |
| THUR | |
| FRI | |
| SAT | |
| SUN | |

# WEEK 13:

### FINE MOTOR

### VISUAL

### AUDITORY

### THIS WEEK'S CHALLENGES

### THIS WEEK'S HIGHLIGHTS

### SOCIAL SKILLS

### OUR FAVORITE MOMENT

# WEEKLY APPOINTMENTS

**WEEK OF:** _____

| MON |
|-----|

_____
_____
_____
_____
_____

| TUE |
|-----|

_____
_____
_____
_____
_____

| WED |
|-----|

_____
_____
_____
_____
_____

| THU |
|-----|

_____
_____
_____
_____

# WEEKLY APPOINTMENTS

**WEEK OF:** _____

FRI

SAT

SUN

# WEEKLY REFLECTION

## Weekly Challenges

## Weekly Accomplishments

## Favorite Moment of the Week

## NOTES

# WEEK 14 ACTIVITIES:

**MONDAY**

**TUESDAY**

**WEDNESDAY**

**THURSDAY**

**FRIDAY**

**SATURDAY**

**SUNDAY**

# WEEK 14:

**WEEK OF:** _____

### SPEECH & COMMUNICATION

### SENSORY & O.T.

### VESTIBULAR

### TACTILE

### ORAL MOTOR

| | |
|---|---|
| MON | |
| TUE | |
| WED | |
| THUR | |
| FRI | |
| SAT | |
| SUN | |

# WEEK 14:

## FINE MOTOR

## VISUAL

## AUDITORY

## THIS WEEK'S CHALLENGES

## SOCIAL SKILLS

## THIS WEEK'S HIGHLIGHTS

## OUR FAVORITE MOMENT

# WEEKLY APPOINTMENTS

**WEEK OF:** _____

MON

TUE

WED

THU

# WEEKLY APPOINTMENTS

**WEEK OF:** _____

FRI

SAT

SUN

# WEEKLY REFLECTION

Weekly Challenges

Weekly Accomplishments

Favorite Moment of the Week

**NOTES**

# WEEK 15 ACTIVITIES:

**MONDAY**

**TUESDAY**

**WEDNESDAY**

**THURSDAY**

**FRIDAY**

**SATURDAY**

**SUNDAY**

# WEEK 15:

**WEEK OF:** _____

## SPEECH & COMMUNICATION

## SENSORY & O.T.

## VESTIBULAR

## TACTILE

## ORAL MOTOR

| | |
|---|---|
| MON | |
| TUE | |
| WED | |
| THUR | |
| FRI | |
| SAT | |
| SUN | |

# WEEK 15:

## FINE MOTOR

## VISUAL

## AUDITORY

## THIS WEEK'S CHALLENGES

## SOCIAL SKILLS

## THIS WEEK'S HIGHLIGHTS

## OUR FAVORITE MOMENT

# WEEKLY APPOINTMENTS

**WEEK OF:** _____

MON

TUE

WED

THU

# WEEKLY APPOINTMENTS

**WEEK OF:** _____

FRI

SAT

SUN

# WEEKLY REFLECTION

Weekly Challenges

Weekly Accomplishments

Favorite Moment of the Week

**NOTES**

# WEEK 16 ACTIVITIES:

**MONDAY**

**TUESDAY**

**WEDNESDAY**

**THURSDAY**

**FRIDAY**

**SATURDAY**

**SUNDAY**

# WEEK 16:

**WEEK OF:** _____

### SPEECH & COMMUNICATION

### SENSORY & O.T.

### VESTIBULAR

### TACTILE

### ORAL MOTOR

| MON | |
|-----|--|
| TUE | |
| WED | |
| THUR | |
| FRI | |
| SAT | |
| SUN | |

# WEEK 16:

## FINE MOTOR

## VISUAL

## AUDITORY

## THIS WEEK'S CHALLENGES

## THIS WEEK'S HIGHLIGHTS

## SOCIAL SKILLS

## OUR FAVORITE MOMENT

# WEEKLY APPOINTMENTS

**WEEK OF:** _____

MON

TUE

WED

THU

# WEEKLY APPOINTMENTS

**WEEK OF:** _____

### FRI

### SAT

### SUN

# WEEKLY REFLECTION

Weekly Challenges

Weekly Accomplishments

Favorite Moment of the Week

## NOTES

# WEEK 17 ACTIVITIES:

**MONDAY**

**TUESDAY**

**WEDNESDAY**

**THURSDAY**

**FRIDAY**

**SATURDAY**

**SUNDAY**

# WEEK 17:

**WEEK OF:** _____

### SPEECH & COMMUNICATION

### SENSORY & O.T.

### VESTIBULAR

### TACTILE

### ORAL MOTOR

| | |
|---|---|
| MON | |
| TUE | |
| WED | |
| THUR | |
| FRI | |
| SAT | |
| SUN | |

# WEEK 17:

## FINE MOTOR

## VISUAL

## AUDITORY

## THIS WEEK'S CHALLENGES

## SOCIAL SKILLS

## THIS WEEK'S HIGHLIGHTS

## OUR FAVORITE MOMENT

# WEEKLY APPOINTMENTS

**WEEK OF:** _____

**MON**

**TUE**

**WED**

**THU**

# WEEKLY APPOINTMENTS

**WEEK OF:** _____

FRI

SAT

SUN

# WEEKLY REFLECTION

## Weekly Challenges

## Weekly Accomplishments

## Favorite Moment of the Week

## NOTES

# WEEK 18 ACTIVITIES:

**MONDAY**

**TUESDAY**

**WEDNESDAY**

**THURSDAY**

**FRIDAY**

**SATURDAY**

**SUNDAY**

# WEEK 18:

**WEEK OF:** _____

## SPEECH & COMMUNICATION

## SENSORY & O.T.

## VESTIBULAR

## TACTILE

## ORAL MOTOR

MON

TUE

WED

THUR

FRI

SAT

SUN

# WEEK 18:

## FINE MOTOR

## VISUAL

## AUDITORY

## THIS WEEK'S CHALLENGES

## SOCIAL SKILLS

## THIS WEEK'S HIGHLIGHTS

## OUR FAVORITE MOMENT

# WEEKLY APPOINTMENTS

**WEEK OF:** _____

MON

_____
_____
_____
_____
_____

TUE

_____
_____
_____
_____

WED

_____
_____
_____
_____

THU

_____
_____
_____
_____

# WEEKLY APPOINTMENTS

**WEEK OF:** _____

| FRI |
|-----|

| SAT |
|-----|

| SUN |
|-----|

# WEEKLY REFLECTION

## Weekly Challenges

## Weekly Accomplishments

## Favorite Moment of the Week

## NOTES

# WEEK 19 ACTIVITIES:

**MONDAY**

**TUESDAY**

**WEDNESDAY**

**THURSDAY**

**FRIDAY**

**SATURDAY**

**SUNDAY**

# WEEK 19:

**WEEK OF:** _____

## SPEECH & COMMUNICATION

## SENSORY & O.T.

## VESTIBULAR

## TACTILE

## ORAL MOTOR

| | |
|---|---|
| MON | |
| TUE | |
| WED | |
| THUR | |
| FRI | |
| SAT | |
| SUN | |

# WEEK 19:

## FINE MOTOR

## VISUAL

## AUDITORY

## THIS WEEK'S CHALLENGES

## THIS WEEK'S HIGHLIGHTS

## SOCIAL SKILLS

## OUR FAVORITE MOMENT

# WEEKLY APPOINTMENTS

**WEEK OF:** _____

**MON**

_____
_____
_____
_____
_____

**TUE**

_____
_____
_____
_____
_____

**WED**

_____
_____
_____
_____
_____

**THU**

_____
_____
_____
_____
_____

# WEEKLY APPOINTMENTS

**WEEK OF:** _____

**FRI**

**SAT**

**SUN**

# WEEKLY REFLECTION

## Weekly Challenges

## Weekly Accomplishments

## Favorite Moment of the Week

## NOTES

# WEEK 20 ACTIVITIES:

MONDAY

TUESDAY

WEDNESDAY

THURSDAY

FRIDAY

SATURDAY

SUNDAY

# WEEK 20:

**WEEK OF:** _____

### SPEECH & COMMUNICATION

### SENSORY & O.T.

### VESTIBULAR

### TACTILE

### ORAL MOTOR

| MON | |
|-----|---|
| TUE | |
| WED | |
| THUR | |
| FRI | |
| SAT | |
| SUN | |

# WEEK 20:

## FINE MOTOR

## VISUAL

## AUDITORY

## THIS WEEK'S CHALLENGES

## SOCIAL SKILLS

## THIS WEEK'S HIGHLIGHTS

## OUR FAVORITE MOMENT

# WEEKLY APPOINTMENTS

**WEEK OF:** _____

**MON**

_____
_____
_____
_____
_____

**TUE**

_____
_____
_____
_____
_____

**WED**

_____
_____
_____
_____
_____

**THU**

_____
_____
_____
_____
_____

# WEEKLY APPOINTMENTS

**WEEK OF:** _____

FRI

SAT

SUN

# WEEKLY REFLECTION

Weekly Challenges

Weekly Accomplishments

Favorite Moment of the Week

**NOTES**

# WEEK 21ACTIVITIES:

**MONDAY**

**TUESDAY**

**WEDNESDAY**

**THURSDAY**

**FRIDAY**

**SATURDAY**

**SUNDAY**

# WEEK 21:

**WEEK OF:** _____

### SPEECH & COMMUNICATION

### SENSORY & O.T.

### VESTIBULAR

### TACTILE

### ORAL MOTOR

| MON |  |
|-----|--|
| TUE |  |
| WED |  |
| THUR |  |
| FRI |  |
| SAT |  |
| SUN |  |

# WEEK 21:

## FINE MOTOR

## VISUAL

## AUDITORY

## THIS WEEK'S CHALLENGES

## SOCIAL SKILLS

## THIS WEEK'S HIGHLIGHTS

## OUR FAVORITE MOMENT

# WEEKLY APPOINTMENTS

**WEEK OF:** _____

**MON**

_____
_____
_____
_____
_____

**TUE**

_____
_____
_____
_____
_____

**WED**

_____
_____
_____
_____
_____

**THU**

_____
_____
_____
_____
_____

# WEEKLY APPOINTMENTS

**WEEK OF:** _____

### FRI

### SAT

### SUN

# WEEKLY REFLECTION

_____
_____
_____
_____
_____
_____
_____
_____
_____
_____
_____
_____
_____
_____
_____
_____
_____
_____
_____
_____
_____

## Weekly Challenges

## Weekly Accomplishments

## Favorite Moment of the Week

## NOTES

# WEEK 22 ACTIVITIES:

**MONDAY**

**TUESDAY**

**WEDNESDAY**

**THURSDAY**

**FRIDAY**

**SATURDAY**

**SUNDAY**

# WEEK 22:

**WEEK OF:** _____

## SPEECH & COMMUNICATION

## SENSORY & O.T.

## VESTIBULAR

## TACTILE

## ORAL MOTOR

| | |
|---|---|
| MON | |
| TUE | |
| WED | |
| THUR | |
| FRI | |
| SAT | |
| SUN | |

# WEEK 22:

### FINE MOTOR

### VISUAL

### AUDITORY

### THIS WEEK'S CHALLENGES

### SOCIAL SKILLS

### THIS WEEK'S HIGHLIGHTS

### OUR FAVORITE MOMENT

# WEEKLY APPOINTMENTS

**WEEK OF:** _____

MON

TUE

WED

THU

# WEEKLY APPOINTMENTS

**WEEK OF:** _____

FRI

SAT

SUN

# WEEKLY REFLECTION

## Weekly Challenges

## Weekly Accomplishments

## Favorite Moment of the Week

**NOTES**

# WEEK 23 ACTIVITIES:

**MONDAY**

**TUESDAY**

**WEDNESDAY**

**THURSDAY**

**FRIDAY**

**SATURDAY**

**SUNDAY**

# WEEK 23:

**WEEK OF:** _____

## SPEECH & COMMUNICATION

## SENSORY & O.T.

## VESTIBULAR

## TACTILE

## ORAL MOTOR

| | |
|---|---|
| **MON** | |
| **TUE** | |
| **WED** | |
| **THUR** | |
| **FRI** | |
| **SAT** | |
| **SUN** | |

# WEEK 23:

## FINE MOTOR

## VISUAL

## AUDITORY

## THIS WEEK'S CHALLENGES

## SOCIAL SKILLS

## THIS WEEK'S HIGHLIGHTS

## OUR FAVORITE MOMENT

# WEEKLY APPOINTMENTS

**WEEK OF:** _____

| MON |
|-----|

_____
_____
_____
_____
_____

| TUE |
|-----|

_____
_____
_____
_____

| WED |
|-----|

_____
_____
_____
_____

| THU |
|-----|

_____
_____
_____
_____

# WEEKLY APPOINTMENTS

**WEEK OF:** _____

**FRI**

**SAT**

**SUN**

# WEEKLY REFLECTION

Weekly Challenges

Weekly Accomplishments

Favorite Moment of the Week

## NOTES

# WEEK 24 ACTIVITIES:

MONDAY

TUESDAY

WEDNESDAY

THURSDAY

FRIDAY

SATURDAY

SUNDAY

# WEEK 24:

**WEEK OF:** _____

## SPEECH & COMMUNICATION

## SENSORY & O.T.

## VESTIBULAR

## TACTILE

## ORAL MOTOR

GOALS & PROGRESS
## TRACKER

| | |
|---|---|
| **MON** | |
| **TUE** | |
| **WED** | |
| **THUR** | |
| **FRI** | |
| **SAT** | |
| **SUN** | |

# WEEK 24:

## FINE MOTOR

## VISUAL

## AUDITORY

## THIS WEEK'S CHALLENGES

## THIS WEEK'S HIGHLIGHTS

## SOCIAL SKILLS

## OUR FAVORITE MOMENT

# WEEKLY APPOINTMENTS

**WEEK OF:** _____

MON

TUE

WED

THU

# WEEKLY APPOINTMENTS

**WEEK OF:** _____

| FRI |
|---|
|  |

| SAT |
|---|
|  |

| SUN |
|---|
|  |

# WEEKLY REFLECTION

| Weekly Challenges |
| --- |
|  |

| Weekly Accomplishments |
| --- |
|  |

| Favorite Moment of the Week |
| --- |
|  |

| NOTES |
| --- |
|  |